Organic Body Scrubs

Easy Homemade Therapeutic Recipes For A Healthy, Youthful And Radiant Skin

PAMELA GODSON

ISBN-13:978-1508506447

ISBN-10:1508506442

DEDICATION

To my beautiful daughters, Maggie and Sue, you make the whole process fun!

TABLE OF CONTENT

INTRODUCTION

Our skin is our body's covering. It is also how other people see us. A dull, lifeless and pre-maturely aged skin brings about insecurity, lack for confidence and ultimately lack of friends. On the contrary, a glowing, healthy skin makes us more youthful, vibrant and assertive.

One sure way to achieve this enviable glow is to do away with chemically-packed skincare products and embrace all-natural, organic beauty products as an increasing number of people have done. And what better place to start than during your bath time with the application of body and face scrubs.

Why Scrub

The main reason for applying body scrub is for exfoliating. Exfoliation is the process of removing dead skin cells that clog up beneath the skin's pore. As humans advance in age, the skin becomes rough and patchy. In exfoliation, the uneven outermost dead layer is removed to reveal a balanced smooth and fresh skin underneath.

Other exfoliation benefits include:

• Removal of excess oil from the skin.

• Increasing blood circulation.

• Reducing the likelihood of blackheads formation and acne breakouts.

• Reducing cellulite.

• Improving the texture of the skin.

• Minimizing wrinkles and fine lines.

• Exposing hair follicle for a closer shave.

• Allowing new cells to regenerate.

• Preparing the skin for an even tan application.

•Removing dull tanned skin.

Applying The Scrubs

The best time to apply scrubs is during a shower or a bath. This is because the still wet skin helps the scrub to spread easily. The surface you are standing or sitting on may become slippery from the scrub's oil so be careful!

When applying body scrubs, gently start from the feet up in an upward circular motion and then move to the legs, arms and then down your back. Finally, move up to your torso. Do not apply to sensitive areas like your pubic areas or nipples. Apply facial scrub gently as you would want to avoid the mouth and eyes. You may want to do this in front of a mirror so you do not make a mistake.

Let the scrub remain on your skin for about 10 minutes to absorb its nutrients and goodness. Afterwards, rinse well with cool water. Do not wipe off the scrub so you do not end up dragging and damaging the skin. You may use a fresh wash cloth instead.

Ensure you thoroughly rinse off and that no residue scrub remains in any part of your body such as the back of your knee or the crook of your arm. Residual sugar, for instance can lead to irritation and yeast infection if it stays in the body for a while.

Gently pat yourself dry without pulling the skin. Finish up this skin pampering experience by applying a good natural moisturizer to your new layer to maximize renewed elasticity and enhance the youthful appearance. There may be slight patches of redness after your scrubs but this will vanish once the new skin layer emerges.

To get the best out of this experience, exfoliate not more than twice a week. Generally, sugar scrubs works for all skin types, which is why most of the scrub recipes in this books are sugar-based. For people with sensitive skin, follow the sugar recipe and instructions in this book to enjoy optimum skin care.

It is also advisable to use a sunscreen when going outside as this protects your newly exposed skin from damage. Nevertheless, do not forget to exfoliate during the winter months as the skin is more prone to the harsh drying weather conditions.

Attaining The Right Texture

If you do not like the texture of the scrub that you have made, you can alter it to suit your preference. All you need is to just change the sugar to oil ratio and use the lighter oil to reduce the quantity of residue.

Nevertheless, the ingredients of homemade scrubs tend to separate after a while, leaving behind a slick of oil on the bathtub or shower tray when the scrub is applied. One way to overcome this issue is to add glycerine to the recipe or replace it with the oil. Glycerine helps to remove the oily residue and bind together the ingredients.

Since glycerin is a very thick and sticky liquid, it is better to replace only half of the oil with it or to rinse really well after a scrub. Additionally, keep the quantities of glycerin in any recipe low because glycerin is powerful humectants. It draws moisture into your skin from the air and has the ability to also draw out moisture from your skin.

Alternately, use a Castile soap, a vegetable- based liquid oil. It is environmentally friendly, completely biodegradable and has no chemical additives. Using a Castile soap adds an element of foaming lather for a rich scrub.

Other Vital Info

For Those With Sensitive Skin

Test the essential oil to be added to the scrub on a tiny and unnoticeable part of your body and let it stay for 24 hours. If no reaction is observed, then it should be safe to use.

You may then proceed to add a new ingredient to the mix and go through the process one more time. Be sure to add the new elements separately so the problem can be traced if you do have a negative reaction.

Some essential oils like cedarwood, lavender and sandalwood are usually better on sensitive skin. If you have a food allergy, you are likely to suffer some form of skin reaction. If you have a nut allergy, for instance, avoid any nut carrier oils. Also, if you are making several batches for friends, make sure you label the jars so they know the things to avoid.

Body Scrubs - Dos And Don'ts

• Do not use body scrubs on damaged or broken skin.

• Do not use glass containers in the bathroom so they don't slip and break, use plastic containers instead.

• Do not allow water to get in your scrubs as it will cause the growth of mold. Store them in air-tight jars in cool, dry places.

• Discard scrubs with rancid smells or visible signs of molds.

BASIC RECIPES

Original Sugar Scrub

Ingredients

2 cups sugar of choice (fine sugar for sensitive face and skin; coarse sugar for a rougher scrub)

1 cup carrier oil of choice

2-3 drops essential oil to suit your skin or mood

Directions

1. Mix all ingredients well.

2. Transfer the now gritty paste to an air tight container using a spoon

3. Label, date and store in a cool place.

4. Use scrub within 3 months.

Basic Sensitive Scrub
- *For people with sensitive skin.*

Ingredients

2 tbsp ground oats

2 tsp brown sugar

2 tbsp aloe Vera

1 tsp almond oil

Directions

1. Grind the rolled oats in a blender until it is a fine powder.

2. Mix all the ingredients into a paste.

Basic Sugar Scrub Cube Recipe
Ingredients

2 parts sugar

1 part melt &pour soap base

1 part carrier oil

Essential oil of choice

Directions

1. Cube the melt& pour soap and then put in a glass jug or bowl.

2. Melt the soap for 20-30 seconds in the microwave and stir.

3. Add essential oil, any preferred coloring, the oil and then mix.

4. Add the sugar, stirring quickly until fully combined. Pour into the mold quickly before it solidifies.

5. The mixture will take about 1 hour to set at room temperature.

6. Once set, just pop out cubes if an ice cube tray was used. If plastic container was used, turn out the block and then cut to the desired size and number of pieces. You can also use a melon baller to make little scrub balls.

7. Keep these individual portions for use or package up a lovely gift.

Simple Whipped Sugar Scrub

<u>Ingredients</u>

1 cup sugar

Vitamin E oil

½ cup carrier oil

1 tbsp water

Essential oils

<u>Directions</u>

1. Put the sugar, water and carrier oil in a bowl and whisk until mixture is light and fluffy.

2. Add essential oils, vitamin E and mix well.

3. Transfer to a wide mouthed jar.

PUNCHY CITRUS SCRUBS

Simple Lemon Sugar Scrub

Ingredients

2 cups white sugar

4 tbsp lemon juice

1 cup extra virgin olive oil

Vitamin E capsule

Directions

1. Mix all ingredients well.

2. Transfer the now gritty paste to an air tight container using a spoon.

3. Label, date and store in a cool place.

4. Use scrub within 3 months.

Lemon& Coconut Milk Scrub

Ingredients

1/4 cup coconut oil

2 tbsp coconut milk

1/4 cup sugar

1 tbsp lemon zest

1 tsp lemon juice

Directions

1. In a double boiler, melt the coconut oil over low heat 15- 20 seconds.

2. Add sugar and coconut milk, mixing until sugar is well coated.

3. Add lemon zest and lemon juice until all ingredients are thoroughly combined.

4. Store in a glass jar.

Organic Citrus Sugar Scrub

<u>Ingredients</u>

1 small lime

1 small lemon

1/2 cup coconut oil

1 cup pure cane sugar

1 teaspoon peppermint essential oil

Mint Leaves, lemon & lime peels (optional)

<u>Directions</u>

1. Mix together the oil and moist ingredients.

2. Add the sugar. If using, add the lime and lemon peels as a garnish.

3. Stir, bottle and use within 3 months.

Citrus Blast Sugar Scrub

<u>Ingredients</u>

1 cup sugar

¼ cup jojoba oil

¼ cup coconut oil

10 drops lemon essential oils

10 drops lime essential oils

10 drops orange essential oils

<u>Directions</u>

1. Mix all ingredients well

2. Transfer the now gritty paste to an air tight container using a spoon

3. Label, date and store in a cool place.

4. Use scrub within 3 months.

Rosemary Lemon Scrub

<u>Ingredients</u>

2 cups white sugar

2 tbsp baking soda

1/4 cup lemon juice

1 cup extra virgin olive oil

1/8 cup rosemary essential oil

1. Combine the ingredients until mixture forms a paste-like substance.

2. Place in a mason jar.

3. Due to the olive oil ingredient, use while showering.

Clementine Coarse Scrub

Ingredients

2 cups turbinado sugar

1 ½ tbsp glycerin

2 tbsp almond oil

1-2 Clementine's rind zest

2 tbsp Clementine juice

Directions

1. Mix all ingredients well

2. Transfer the now gritty paste to an air tight container using a spoon

3. Label, date and store in a cool place.

4. Use scrub within 3 months.

Orange Sugar Scrub
<u>Ingredients</u>

3/4 cup sugar (plus 1-2tbsp more)

4 drops orange essential oil

1/4 cup coconut oil (melted)

1 tbsp dried orange peel (coarsely grinded)

1/4 cup olive oil

<u>Directions:</u>

1. Mix all ingredients together and place it in a clean container.

2. If mixture is too dry, add some more oil. If too oily, add a little more sugar.

Lime Margarita Mousse Scrub

<u>Ingredients</u>

2 drops lemon essential oil

4 drops lime essential oil

½ tsp lime or lemon juice

2 tsp virgin coconut oil

1½ tsp salt

2 tsp white sugar

10 drops kukui nut oil, sweet almond oil or apricot kernel oil

<u>Directions</u>

1. Combine the ingredients well.

2. (The salt will stay nice and grainy but the sugar will mostly dissolve in the lime juice)

3. Apply to body.

Lemon Poppy Seed Scrub

Ingredients

2 ½ cups raw sugar

Juice of 2 lemons

1 tsp poppy seeds

1 cup olive oil

Directions

1. Mix ingredients up.

2. Put it in a jar.

3. Apply to hands and say goodbye to those dry hands.

OATMEAL SCRUBS

Simple Oatmeal Scrub

Ingredients

1 tbsp oatmeal

3 tbsp warm water or more

Directions

1. Combine ingredients.

2. Wait for about 10 minutes until oats soften and then use.

Spicy Oat Scrub

Ingredients

1/2 cup oats

1/2 cup brown rice

1/4 cup oregano (dried)

1/4 cup comfrey (dried)

1/2 cup calendula

1/4 cup myrrh

1/8 cup anise seed

1 1/2 cups clay

1 drop lavender essential oil

1 drop tea tree essential oil

Directions

1. Grind all ingredients except oils until powdery.

2. Add oils and then stir well.

3. Store in a jar.

4. To use: combine 1-2 tsp scrub and add a small amount of water.

Seedy Oatmeal Body Scrub

Ingredients

1 handful coarse rolled oats

1 handful brown lentils

1/2 tsp jojoba oil

1/2 tsp carrot oil

Water

<u>Directions</u>

1. Blend the lentils in a blender until it is a coarse powder.

2. Add the rolled oats and blend to make powder. Add the oils and then process again.

3. Add water a teaspoon at a time until mixture becomes a thick paste.

4. Spoon into a container.

Oats & Coffee Body Scrub
<u>Ingredients</u>

1/3 cup rolled oats, chopped

2 tsp coffee grounds

2 tsp raw honey

2 tbsp coconut oil

<u>Directions:</u>

1. Combine all the ingredients in a bowl, mixing well.

Coconut Oatmeal Scrub

Ingredients

1/2 cup organic coconut oil

1 1/2 cup oatmeal

1 tsp brown sugar

1 tsp vanilla extract

1 tsp honey

Directions

1. In a food processor, ground oatmeal and place in a bowl.

2. Add brown sugar to finely ground oatmeal and then mix.

3. Pour vanilla, coconut oil and honey to the oatmeal and then mix until thoroughly combined.

4. Store in an airtight container.

Cucumber Oatmeal Scrub

<u>Ingredients</u>

1 cucumber (2 tbsp cucumber paste)

1tsp rosehip oil

1 teaspoon argan oil

2 tbsp oatmeal

1 tbsp milk

<u>Directions</u>

1. Blend cucumber in the blender to make a paste.

2. Add 2 tablespoon of the blended cucumber with the rest of the ingredients, mixing well.

3. Leave for about 5 minutes until oatmeal gets soft.

4. Use and discard leftover.

Milky Oatmeal Scrub

<u>Ingredients</u>

1 tbsp whole milk

1 tbsp extra virgin olive oil

1 tbsp honey

2 tbsp oatmeal

Directions

1. Combine ingredients in a bowl.

2. Leave for 5 to 10 minutes and then use.

Oatmeal & Brown Sugar Scrub
A quick and gentle facial scrub

Ingredients

2 tsp brown sugar

2 tbsp fine colloidal oatmeal fine

1 tsp citrus blend floral water

2 tbsp aloe moist

Directions

1. Combine ingredients in a bowl until a smooth pasties achieved

SUGAR SCRUBS FOR SPECIFIC BODY AREAS

Vanilla Sugar Lip Scrub

Ingredients

1 tbsp fine sugar

Drop vanilla essential oil

1 tsp jojoba oil

Directions

1. Mix all ingredients well

2. Transfer the now gritty paste to an air tight container using a spoon

3. Label, date and store in a cool place.

Lemon Face Sugar Scrub

<u>Ingredients</u>

½ cup fine sugar

½ juice of lemon

1 tbsp honey

1 tbsp evening primrose oil

<u>Directions</u>

1. Combine all the ingredients so it forms a paste.

2. Use a spoon to transfer mixture to an air -tight jar.

3. Label jar, date and store it in a cool and place.

4. Use within 3 months.

Yogurt Sugar Face Mask

<u>Ingredients</u>

2 tsp sugar

3 tsp plain yogurt

<u>Directions</u>

1. Combine all the ingredients so it forms a paste.

2. Use a spoon to transfer mixture to an air -tight jar.

3. Use and discard any left. Do not store.

Citrus Lavender Hand Scrub

<u>Ingredients</u>

1 tbsp dried lavender

⅓ Cup olive oil

2 tsp lemon zest

1 cup kosher salt

1 tbsp lemon juice from 1 small lemon (freshly squeezed)

<u>Directions</u>

1. In a small pan over low heat, place the lavender and olive oil to warm for about 5 minutes.

2. Turn heat off and allow the infused oil cool to room temperature.

3. Combine salt, lemon juice and lemon zest in a small bowl.

4. Stir in the infused oil

5. Transfer scrub to a glass jar with an airtight lid and then store.

Peppermint Foot Sugar Scrub
<u>Ingredients</u>

1 cup turbinado sugar

1 tsp. peppermint essential oil

½ cup jojoba oil

<u>Directions</u>

1. Mix all ingredients really well until mixture forms a paste.

2. Spoon into a glass container with a lid that seals.

3. Use the scrub within a couple of months.

Sugar Cookie Foot Scrub
<u>Ingredients</u>

1/3 cup packed brown sugar

2/3 cup granulated white sugar

1 tbsp vanilla extract

1/2 cup olive oil

Directions

1. Combine white sugar & brown sugar in a medium sized bowl.

2. Whisk together until well combined.

3. Add olive oil and vanilla extract and then use a fork to mash together until the oil is incorporated into the sugar mixture.

4. Pack the mixture into an air tight jar.

5. Label, date and store in a cool place.

Gardener's Hand Sugar Scrub

Ingredients

1 cup sugar

½ tsp vitamin E

½ cup almond oil

1 tsp lavender

Directions

1. Mix all ingredients really well until mixture forms a paste.

2. Spoon into a glass container with a lid that seals.

3. Use the scrub within a couple of months.

COFFEE CUP SCRUBS

Coffee Morning Scrub

Ingredients

2 tbsp freshly ground coffee

3 tbsp whole milk or heavy cream

2 tbsp cocoa powder

1 tbsp honey

Directions:

1. Mix all together and apply lightly to face.

2. Leave for 15-20 minutes.

3. Remove with warm wash cloth.

Get Up & Go Scrub

<u>Ingredients</u>

1 cup turbinado sugar

1 cup ground coffee

2 tbsp coconut oil

1 tbsp jojoba oil

1 tsp ginger essential oil

<u>Directions</u>

1. Mix all ingredients well

2. Transfer the now gritty paste to an air tight container using a spoon

3. Label, date and store in a cool place.

4. Use scrub within 3 months.

Coconut Coffee Scrub

Ingredients

1/2 cup ground coffee

1/4 cup coconut oil

1/2 cup coconut palm sugar

1 tsp ground cinnamon

Directions

1. Mix together all ingredients until well-combined.

2. If coconut oil is solid, heat gently until it melts and then let it return to room temperature before adding other ingredients.

3. Once mixed, store in an air-tight container.

Anti-Cellulite Coffee Scrub

Ingredients

½ cup ground coffee

1 ½ cup turbinado sugar

½ cup grape seed oil

½ cup jojoba oil

1 tsp vitamin E

1 tsp vanilla extract

1 tsp sage essential oil

Directions

1. Mix all ingredients well

2. Transfer the now gritty paste to an air tight container using a spoon

3. Label, date and store in a cool place.

4. Use scrub within 3 months.

Cup Of Joe Scrub

Ingredients

6 tbsp coffee grounds

1/3 cup brown sugar

4 tbsp olive oil

Directions

1. Mix the two ingredients together until it looks like a coarse mud.

2. (The coffee grounds have to be very fine as they will be rubbed onto the skin. If necessary, put them through a coffee grinder twice)

3. Transfer to a container, refrigerate or store at room temperature for 5-7 weeks.

Citrus Coffee Scrub

<u>Ingredients</u>

1 cup coconut oil, melted

1 cup coffee grounds

1-3 drops orange essential oil

1-3 drops lemon essential oil

½ cup coconut sugar

<u>Directions</u>

1. Mix all ingredients in a bowl until thoroughly.

2. Keep at room temperature, use and store leftover in a mason jar.

Coffee Sugar Scrub

Ingredients

1/2 cup used ground coffee

1/2 cup ground coffee

1/2 cup coconut oil

1 cup sugar

1 tsp cinnamon

1 tsp vegetable glycerin (for extra moisturizer)

Directions

1. Pour coffee grounds and sugar into a medium sized bowl.

2. Stir in coconut oil or more if you prefer a wet consistency.

3. Now add cinnamon, mix and place in the jar.

Vitalizing Pumpkin Coffee Scrub

Ingredients

1/2 cup brown sugar

2 tbsp ground coffee beans

2 tbsp extra virgin olive oil

1/2 cup canned pumpkin

2 tbsp fresh lemon juice

Directions

1. In a medium sized bowl, combine all the ingredients and spoon into a jar.

2. Use and refrigerate leftover for 3 to 4 days

WARMING WINTER SCRUBS

Christmas Scent Sugar Scrub

Ingredients

1 cup brown sugar

1 cup white sugar

½ cup glycerin

1 tsp ground cloves

½ cup cocoa butter oil

½ tsp ground cinnamon

1 tsp ground nutmeg

Directions

1. Combine all the ingredients in a jar, mixing well.

2. Label, date and store in a cool place.

3. Use within a couple of months.

Magnesium Winter Scrub

Ingredients

1 cup Epsom salt

¼ cup almond oil or olive oil

1 tsp liquid castile soap

10-15 drops peppermint and citrus essential oils

Directions

1. Mix all ingredients together in a small bowl.

2. Add essential oils until desired fragrance is achieved.

3. Store in an airtight jar.

4. Use a teaspoon sized amount to exfoliate body as needed.

5. Rinse after use.

6. Use within 3 months.

Spicy Sugar Scrub

Ingredients

1 cup sugar

2 tsp ground cloves

1 cup sesame oil

1 tsp rose essential oil

2 tsp grated orange zest

Directions

1. Mix all ingredients well.

2. Transfer the now gritty paste to an air tight container using a spoon.

3. Label, date and store in a cool place.

4. Use scrub within 3 months.

Warming Gingerbread Scrub

<u>Ingredients</u>

1 cup of vegetable glycerin

1/3 cup of olive oil

2 cups dark brown sugar

1 cup turbinado sugar

1/3 cup cocoa butter

1 tablespoon spoon or more of gingerbread fragrance oil

 5 drops of liquipar oil

<u>Directions</u>

1. Combine all the ingredients in a plastic bowl, mixing well.

 2. Transfer to wide mouth jars.

Spicy Pumpkin Ginger Scrub

<u>Ingredients</u>

1/2 cup canned pumpkin

1 tbsp fresh lemon juice

2 tbsp fresh ginger, grated

1/2 cup demerara sugar or any coarse sugar

1 tbsp extra virgin olive oil

1 tbsp ground cinnamon

<u>Directions</u>

1. In a medium sized bowl, combine all the ingredients and spoon into a jar.

2. Use on feet and refrigerate leftover for 3 to 4 days.

Chocó Mocha Scrub

<u>Ingredients</u>

1 cup sugar

1 tbsp ground coffee

½ cup macadamia nut oil

1 tsp cinnamon

1 tbsp cocoa powder

½ tsp nutmeg

<u>Directions</u>

1. Combine all the ingredients so it forms a paste.

2. Use a spoon to transfer mixture to an air -tight jar.

3. Label jar, date and store it in a cool and place.

Preferred Spice Sugar Scrub

<u>Ingredients</u>

½ cup brown sugar

½ cup turbinado sugar

¼ cup almond oil

¼ cup coconut oil

1 tsp pumpkin or apple pie spice

<u>Directions</u>

1. Combine all the ingredients so it forms a paste.

2. Use a spoon to transfer mixture to an air -tight jar.

3. Label jar, date and store it in a cool and place.

Soothing Brown Sugar Scrub

<u>Ingredients</u>

1 cup brown sugar

½ tsp rosewood essential oil

½ cup almond oil

½ tsp lavender essential oil

<u>Directions</u>

1. Mix all the ingredients together until it is paste-like.

2. Transfer to an air -tight container.

3. Store it in a cool and place.

CUBES AND WHIPPED SUGAR SCRUBS

Brown Sugar Scrub Cubes

Ingredients

1 cup brown sugar

1 tsp honey

½ cup avocado oil

½ cup melted melt & pour soap

1 tsp essential oil

Directions

1. Mix all ingredients well.

2. Transfer the now gritty paste to an air tight container using a spoon

3. Label, date and store in a cool place.

4. Use scrub within 3 months.

Vanilla Whipped Sugar Scrub

Ingredients

1 cup sugar

½ tsp vanilla extract

½ cup jojoba oil

Directions

1. Combine all ingredients and whisk until thick and creamy.

Whipped Shea Butter Scrub

Ingredients

1 cup sugar

¼ cup almond oil

½ cup Shea butter

½ tsp. vitamin E oil

Directions

1. Put the Shea butter in the microwave to soften.

2. Using a mixer, whisk until thick and creamy.

3. Gradually add the almond oil in stages, mixing well between each addition.

4. Now, add vitamin E and then mix thoroughly.

5. Gradually add the sugar in stages, mixing until the desired consistency is attained.

Solid Shea Butter Cube

Ingredients

4 oz refined Shea butter

2.5 oz Shea butter soap base

2 tbsp fractionated coconut oil

16 oz white sugar

½ tbsp essential oils of choice

Pinch of mica (optional)

Directions

1. Weigh out the melt and pour soap base then melt. Weigh out Shea butter and melt.

2. Add the Shea butter into the melt & pour soap base and stir. Add the fractionated coconut oil and essential oils and stir.

3. Pour the sugar into the soap/ Shea mixture, mixing well. Scoop into mold and use a spatula to level. Refrigerate until solidified.

4. Remove the scrub gently from the molds. Remove plastic wrap from scrub. Cut the scrub into cubes with a Chef's knife.

5. Place cubes in an airtight jar until use.

Whipped Super Shea Butter Scrub

Ingredients

1/2 cup raw Shea butter

1/3 cup apricot kernel or sweet almond

1/8 tsp rosemary extract

1 tsp corn starch (to make the butter feel less greasy)

2-3 drops grapefruit or rosemary essential oil (optional)

1/2 –1 cup sugar

Directions

1. Place Shea butter in a mixing bowl and then beat until the butter is creamy.

2. If butter is too hard, put in the microwave to soften for 15 seconds but don't melt.

3. Add the carrier oil a little at a time and blend fully between additions.

4. Add the rosemary extract and then the cornstarch and essential oil, blending well.

5. Mix in the sugar gradually until the desired consistency is achieved.

DELICIOUS VANILLA SCRUBS

Cinnamon Vanilla Body Scrub

Ingredients

1/2-3/4 cup raw sugar

1 cup brown sugar

2 tbsp raw honey

1/2 cup sea salt

1/4 cup coconut oil (liquefy if solid)

1/2 cup avocado oil

1 tsp cinnamon

1-2 tsp vanilla extract

1 tsp freshly grated nutmeg (optional)

5 drops nutmeg essential oil

5 drops cinnamon essential oil

Directions

1. Combine the salt and sugars.

2. Add avocado oil, vanilla extract, essential oils and spice(s).

3. Add to 2 half pint jars and enjoy!

Simple Vanilla Sugar Scrub

<u>Ingredients</u>

½ cup brown sugar

½ cup white sugar

1 tsp. vanilla essential oil

½ cup grape seed oil

<u>Directions</u>

1. Mix all ingredients well.

2. Transfer the now gritty paste to an air tight container using a spoon.

3. Label, date and store in a cool place.

4. Use immediately.

Scented Vanilla Scrub

<u>Ingredients</u>

1 cup sugar

1 cup grape seed oil

½ cup salt

1 tbsp lemon or mint essential oils

<u>Directions</u>

1. Combine all of these ingredients well.

2. Transfer the now gritty paste to an air tight container using a spoon.

3. Label and store.

Vanilla Banana Scrub

<u>Ingredients</u>

1 cup sugar

1 ripe banana mashed

1 tsp vanilla essential oil

¼ cup jojoba oil

1. Mash the banana lightly using a fork.

2. Combine with ingredients until it forms a thick paste.

3. Use immediately.

Vanilla Chamomile Scrub

Ingredients

1 cup sugar

¼ cup honey

½ cup jojoba oil

1 tsp chamomile essential oil

1 tsp vanilla essential oil

Directions

1. Mix all ingredients well.

2. Transfer the now gritty paste to an air tight container using a spoon.

3. Label and store.

Soothing Vanilla Sugar Scrub

<u>Ingredients</u>

1 cup fine sugar

1 tbsp honey

½ cup almond oil

½ tsp vanilla

1 tsp vitamin E

<u>Directions</u>

1. Combine all the ingredients so it forms a paste.

2. Use a spoon to transfer mixture to an air-tight jar.

3. Label jar, date and store it in a cool and place.

HONEY SCRUBS

Honey Sesame Scrub

<u>Ingredients</u>

2 cup sugar

1 tbsp honey

1 cup sesame oil

½ tbsp lemon juice

<u>Directions</u>

1. Mix all ingredients well.

2. Transfer the now gritty paste to an air tight container using a spoon.

3. Label and store.

Honey Chamomile Scrub

<u>Ingredients</u>

1 cup sugar

2 tbsp chamomile essential oil

½ cup honey

Directions

1. Mix all ingredients well.

2. Transfer the now gritty paste to an air tight container using a spoon

3. Label, date and store in a cool place.

4. Use scrub within 3 months.

Brown Sugar Honey Scrub

<u>Ingredients</u>

1 tbsp raw honey

1 tbsp brown sugar

<u>Directions</u>

1. In a small bowl, place the honey and brown sugar and mix well.

2. Store in a container with an air tight lid.

3. Wash face and apply about ½ tsp to wet skin.

4. Gently massage in a circular motion. Keep away from eye area.

5. Rinse face and pat dry.

Honey Coffee Body Scrub
Ingredients

1/2 cup very finely ground coffee

3 tbsp honey

1/4 cup brown sugar

1 tbsp vanilla extract

2 tbsp olive oil

Directions

1. Combine ingredients well.

2. Store for up to 1 month in an airtight container.

Simple Honey Sugar Scrub
Ingredients

1 cup sugar

1 tsp pure honey

¼ cup jojoba oil

½ tsp ylang ylang essential oil

½ tsp orange essential oil

Directions

1. Mix all ingredients well.

2. Transfer the now gritty paste to an air tight container using a spoon.

3. Label and store.

MINTY FRESH SCRUB RECIPES

Mint Eucalyptus Scrub
For the feet

<u>Ingredients</u>

2 cup fine or medium ground sea salt (for rougher feet, use coarser salt)

1 cup coconut oil

15 drops peppermint essential oil

25 drops eucalyptus essential oil

<u>Directions</u>

1. Combine all the ingredients in a jar.

2. Apply scrub with bare hands or wash cloths.

3. Scrub feet gently until smooth and supple and then rinse.

Peppermint Sugar Scrub

<u>Ingredients</u>

2 cups sugar

½ cup honey

1 tsp peppermint essential oil

¼ cup almond oil

<u>Directions</u>

1. Mix all ingredients well.

2. Transfer the now gritty paste to an air tight container using a spoon.

3. Label and store.

Peppermint Citrus Scrub

For dry, itchy skin

<u>Ingredients</u>

1 cup granulated white sugar

10 drops peppermint essential oil

1/4-1/3 cup olive, avocado or apricot oil or a combination

2-4 tbsp orange or grapefruit zest (for extra exfoliation)

2 tbsp vegetable glycerin (extra moisturizing)

10-15 drops wild orange or grapefruit essential oil

<u>Directions</u>

1. Mix together sugar, zest, oil and vegetable glycerin.

2. Gently add essential oils until the desired scent is reached.

3. Store in a glass container.

Rosemary Mint Sugar Scrub
<u>Ingredients</u>

2 cups sugar

1 cup coconut oil

1 tsp peppermint essential oil

1 tsp rosemary essential oil

1. Combine all the ingredients so it forms a paste.

2. Use a spoon to transfer mixture to an air -tight jar.

3. Label jar, date and store it in a cool and place.

Mint Salt Scrub Recipe

This moisturizing scrub doubles as soap

Ingredients

3/8 cup Epsom salts

1/8 cup liquid castile soap

1/2 oz glycerin soap base

1 tbsp jojoba oil

1/8 cup sunflower or safflower oil

4 drops peppermint essential oil

2 drops tea tree essential oil

1 tsp aloe gel (optional)

Green or blue mica powder for color (optional)

Directions

1. Melt the glycerin soap base.

2. Add oils and liquid soap. Remove from heat.

3. Add essential oils, salt, aloe and color. (Mix the powder with some oil before you mix it in).

4. Plop the now thick mixture into a plastic or glass container. Let it cool.

Peppermint Candy Cane Scrub

Ingredients

4 tbsp plus 2 tsp granulated sugar

3-4 drops peppermint essential oil

2 tbsp extra virgin olive oil

1 teaspoon flax seed oil

Directions

1. Add together all of the ingredients, stirring well.

2. Sugar usually settles at the bottom so shake before using.

SCRUB RECIPES WITH NUTS

Almond Sugar Scrub

Ingredients

1 cup turbinado sugar

1 cup sugar

1 tsp vitamin E

1 cup almond oil

Directions

1. Combine all of these ingredients thoroughly until it forms a paste.

2. Transfer to a container.

3. Label the container and store it in a cool and dark place.

4. Shelf life: 2-3 months.

Vanilla Almond Scrub

Ingredients

3 parts brown sugar

2 parts sweet almond oil

1 cup oats

1 teaspoon almond extract

Handful of almonds

2-3 drops essential oil of choice (optional)

Directions

1. Mix all the ingredients in a food processor.

2. Apply to body

Apricot Kernel Scrub

Ingredients

1.5 oz ground apricot kernel

2 oz orange blossom floral water or citrus blend

1 oz aloe Vera gel

1 oz melt & pour glycerin soap

1 drop sandalwood essential oil

2 drop orange essential oil

1 oz rice bran oil

Safflower oil

<u>Directions</u>

1. Melt the soap in a double boiler. Add the safflower oil and aloe Vera gel.

2. Remove from heat; add the floral water and essential oils, mixing thoroughly. Add ground apricot kernel and stir frequently.

3. Let the mixture cool. Scrape the scrub into containers and seal for 1-2 days for ingredients to blend. Apply.

Nutty Sugar Scrub

<u>Ingredients</u>

1 cup sugar

½ cup ground oatmeal

½ cup macadamia nut oil

½ cup ground almonds

½ cup almond oil

1 tsp Neroli essential oil

Directions

1. Mix all ingredients well.

2. Transfer the now gritty paste to an air tight container using a spoon

3. Label, date and store in a cool place.

4. Use scrub within 3 months.

Honey Almond Sleepy Sugar Scrub

<u>Ingredients</u>

3 parts white sugar

1 part honey

2 tbsp tea

1 tsp almond extract

<u>Directions</u>

1. Mix all ingredients well. Ensure that it is not lumpy or break apart.

2. Transfer to a jar and use.

Almond Oatmeal Facial Scrub Recipe
Ingredients

1/4 cup almonds

1/4 cup oatmeal

1 tbsp cornstarch

1 tbsp chamomile flower tea (optional)

Directions

1. Add all the ingredients to a blender or food processor and process until the mixture looks like a fine mealy-textured powder.

2. Transfer to small glass jars.

OTHERS

Aloe Vera Scrub

<u>Ingredients</u>

1 cup fine sugar

2 tbsp aloe Vera gel

1 tsp chamomile essential oil

1 cup calendula oil

<u>Directions</u>

1. Mix all ingredients well

2. Transfer the now gritty paste to an air tight container using a spoon

3. Label, date and store in a cool place.

Chocolate Marshmallow Scrub

Good for dry skin

<u>Ingredients</u>

4 oz. Shea butter

4 oz. cocoa butter

4 oz. fractionated coconut oil

2 tbsp Natrasorb

1 1/4 cup turbinado sugar

1/4 cup dendritic salt

1 tsp polysorbate 20

1 tsp milk chocolate fragrance oil

1 tbsp marshmallow root powder

1 tbsp milk powder

1 tbsp cocoa powder

<u>Directions</u>

1. Heat the oils and butters until melted.

2. Blend the additives, Natrasorb and powders in a separate bowl.

3. Mix the polysorbate 20 and fragrance and add to the Natrasorb.

4. Now add the turbinado sugar, mix well and gently pour oil over the sugar blend.

5. Let the mixture cool. Store and use at room temperature.

White Chocolate &Strawberries Scrub
Ingredients

1 cup turbinado or demerara sugar

1 oz strawberry seed oil

 2 oz cocoa butter

20 drops strawberry fragrance oil

1 tbsp strawberry seeds

Directions

1. Melt the cocoa butter and add the strawberry oil.

2. Mix together all dry ingredients and stir.

3. Pour oil mixture over dry mixture, stirring well.

Totally Herbal Body Exfoliant

<u>Ingredients</u>

1/2 cup Norwegian kelp powder

1/2 cup bladderwrack powder

1/3 cup of Dead Sea clay

1/2 cup Dead Sea salt

1/2 cup walnut oil

1/3 cup of emu oil

1 cup jojoba oil

10 drops of liquipar oil

1 tablespoon T-50 vitamin E oil

<u>Directions</u>

1. Combine ingredients in a large bowl and then mix thoroughly.

2. If mixture is too wet, add more clay and if too dry, add more emu oil until it is a little slushy.

Cleansing Aromatic Salt Glow

<u>Ingredients:</u>

1/4 cup Epsom salts

1/4 cup sea salt

1 tbsp borax

1/4 cup almond oil

1 tbsp baking soda

8 drops geranium essential oil

4 drops lavender essential oil

<u>Directions</u>

1. Mix salts in canning jar. Add borax and baking soda and mix again.

2. Add the essential oils to almond oil then mix with salts mixture.

3. Add the oils to the mixture and then mix well and store.

Lemon Milk Sugar Scrub

1 cup sugar

¼ cup milk

2 tbsp olive oil

4 drops lemon essential oil

Juice from one lemon

<u>Directions</u>

1. Mix all ingredients well

2. Transfer the now gritty paste to an air tight container using a spoon

3. Label, date and store in a cool place.

4. Use immediately.